I0844917

TABLE OF CONTENTS

What Is Smarter Eating?

A lot of our foods are loaded with unnecessarily high amounts of calories in order to maximize taste or to make recipes easier to make.

But we can change the recipes to reduce calories or make the food less calorie dense while retaining most of that taste. Is it going to be a perfect 10 out of 10? No. But if it's still an 8 out of 10 but is more filling and helps you control your weight is that really such a bad thing?

Even when we eat out, by picking the right things off the menu and by making substitutions we can better control our eating with minimal effect on how good it tastes.

Enjoying What You Eat

In order for a diet to be successful you need to enjoy your food. Forcing yourself to eat things you don't like will never be sustainable.

Too many diets are unsuccessful because we want weight loss so bad that we force ourselves to eat this magic diet that cuts out food we love, and after a year of that you want to go back to eating the food you love! And I don't blame you, if I had to eat something I didn't like for a year I'd for sure over-eat the things I love the instant I came back to them.

Stop cutting out the foods you love, start making changes to them to reduce calories while still being able to eat them.

<u>Rules To Cook By</u>

1. Egg whites are a great way to add protein. They are literally just amino acids floating in water. They also don't contain animal cells and are vegetarian.

2. Whenever possible, just drop the oil or butter out of a recipe. Most of the time it's just added for a little extra flavour but comes at the cost of 100 calories.

3. Cooking sprays are 10 calories per second of spray, not 0 calories. Use a quick spritz and just use some paper towel to spread it around.

4. It's okay to replace sugar with artificial sweetener.

5. It's also okay to replace part of the flour in a recipe with protein powder.

6. It's perfectly okay to buy packaged or frozen foods, just as long as they aren't packed in oil (example: buy canned tuna packed in water not oil).

<u>What's Best To Order When Eating Out</u>

When eating at fast food places, it's best to avoid mayo and sauces which tend to be very high fat, highly caloric dense. Ketchup is "okay", it's usually a bit sugary but still better than mayo. Mustard is amazing and perfectly fine.

You want to avoid the fries, you're getting enough carbs from the bun and breading. If you really want fries, swap the burger bun for a lettuce wrap instead.

Always ask for triple lettuce! It usually costs nothing extra and makes the meal that much less calorie dense.

A&W

- 5pc Chicken Tenders

- Chicken Club Sandwich

- Chicken Sandwich

- Plain Hamburger

- Cheeseburger

Arby's

- Roast Turkey Gyro

- Any wrap or salad

- Classic Roast Chicken

- Roast Buffalo Chicken

- Chicken Tenders with BBQ or Buffalo sauce

- Classic Roast Beef

- Double Roast Beef

- Half Pound Roast Beef

Burger King

- Plain burger, everything else is super fatty, even the chicken

Chick-Fil-A

- All of their chicken entrees are fine

- Egg White Grill

- Chicken, Egg & Cheese Bagel

Dairy Queen

- *The chicken salads. I'd just avoid Dairy Queen to be honest.*

KFC

- *Any grilled chicken option. If your KFC doesn't have grilled chicken, I recommend avoiding KFC, their chicken is super fatty.*

McDonald's

- *Plain Hamburger*
- *Cheeseburger*
- *Keep Calm, Caesar On Salad with Grilled Chicken*

Popeye's

- *Bonafide Chicken Breast + one other (breast, leg, wing, thigh)*
- *Chicken Sandwich*

Subway

- BBQ Chicken
- Buffalo Chicken
- Chicken Mango Curry
- Chicken Tikka
- Chicken Vindaloo
- Oven Roasted Chicken
- Roast Beef
- Rotisserie-Style Chicken
- Steak & Cheese
- Subway Club
- Turkey & Bacon
- Turkey Breast
- Turkey Breast & Black Forest Ham
- Turkey Reuben

Taco Bell

- Chicken Burrito Supreme
- Steak Burrito Supreme
- Chicken Soft Taco

Wendy's

- Grilled Chicken Sandwich
- Homestyle Chicken Sandwich
- Spicy Chicken Sandwich
- Chicken Wraps

At The Pancake Place

- You have a choice, you can have egg yolks or bacon, don't get both. If you want bacon then order egg whites only. If you want egg yolks, get turkey bacon if available.

- Two words: Grilled. Ham.

- Sausages are all fat, stick to the ham.

- Having a pancake is fine. Having a stack of six pancakes is a no.

- Build your own omelette – Egg white, ham and veggies. You can even have some cheese that's such a good combo.

At The Pizza Parlour

- Stick with personal or small size, you don't need a large to yourself

- Ask for half cheese, and if available ask for the other half to be low-fat cheese

- Don't be afraid to get double meat and double veggies on your pizza, those are the parts you want

- You can also ask them to serve the pizza on a bed of napkins or paper bags to soak up some of the fats

At The Restaurant

- *Unless you know how lean the beef or pork cut is, stick with chicken or fish dishes*

- *Ask for half the starchy carb (rice, potatoes, etc) and twice the vegetable side*

- *If you go to a smorgasbord with family or friends, order off the menu so you aren't encouraged to eat multiple plates*

- *Just avoid anything fried, there's so many better choices on the menu*

At The Bar

- *Oven Baked Shrimp is the perfect bar snack*

- *Don't be afraid to sneak in a protein bar*

- *Don't touch the bar nuts! Not only are nuts highly calorie dense but they're loaded with salt to encourage you to drink more.*

Sweeteners

Cyclamate – Is the primary artificial sweetener I use, it has a slightly salty taste to it which works great with cooking and baking, but may not taste well in coffee, tea or glazes depending on personal taste preferences. It is also one of the cheapest per packet.

One Packet = 1/4 tsp

Brands: Sugar Twin, Sweet'N'Low (Canada only)

Sucralose – I keep on hand for recipes where cyclamate doesn't taste as good. It's slightly weaker than cyclamate and costs nearly twice as much, but doesn't have the salty taste to it.

One Packet = 1/4 tsp

Brands: Splenda

Erythritol – Is a sugar alcohol that is 70% as sweet as sugar for a fraction of the calories and mixes well into a sugar syrup form. However over consumption of sugar alcohols can lead to bloating or even diarrhea, so I limit it to just in use of icing where it shines best.

Brands: Swerve, NOW Foods

Stevia – I do not like the taste of stevia and so it won't be found in any recipes. I have no idea how it will taste if you replace sweeteners in any recipes with stevia but you are welcome to try if stevia is your sweetener of choice.

Recommended Low Calorie Toppings

Fish Sauce

Frank's Hot Sauce

Guy's BBQ Sauce

Heinz No Sugar Added Ketchup

Kraft Fat Free Italian Dressing

Mrs Butterworth Sugar Free Maple Syrup

Mustard

Popcorn Seasonings

Smucker's Sugar Free Jam

Skinny Sauce

St. Hubert Dijon Gravy

Tostitos Salsa

Walden Farms Chocolate Sauce

Walden Farms Mocha Creamer

Water Enhancers eg Mio (not just for water, can be used on yogurt for example)

Worcestershire Sauce

Good Prepackaged Snacks

- Protein Bars (Pure Protein brand bars are just over $1 per bar, you don't need $4 Quest bars)

- Flavoured Egg White Drink (Liquid Muscle, MuscleEgg)

- Rule 1 Easy Protein Mousse

- Nutraphase Clean Beans

- The Smart Co Smart Tart

- MHP Power Pak Pudding

- Twin Peak Ingredients Protein Puffs

- IWON Organics Protein Stix

- IWON Organics Protein Chips

- Optimum Nutrition Protein Ridges

- Quest Nutrition Tortilla Chips

- Flapjacked Mighty Muffin

Vegan Egg White Replacers

Vegg - Power Scramble

Just Egg

Just Egg Folded

Egg Whites

IMPORTANT

Recipes assume use of pasteurized egg whites from cartons. If you're using egg whites from eggs in recipes that are not cooked you will need to pasteurize them yourself first to avoid salmonella.

Recipe Serving Sizes

Recipes were written with single serving size in mind whenever possible. This makes it extremely easy to make a single serving and know approximately how many calories you ate.

In order to make bigger servings for multiple people or for meal prep, simply multiply the ingredients by the amount of servings you want to make. Or just make multiple individual servings separately.

> **Vegan Version**
> Most vegan version changes will result in slightly lower protein totals (and slightly less overall calories).
>
> If you're a vegan and you feel your calories or protein intake are too low, I recommend adding a 200 calorie high protein snack to your day, either from this book or from the nutrition guide!

ANABOLIC MILK

Anabolic Milk (Cake Batter)

Ingredients

1 cup Egg White
1 tsp Vanilla Extract
1 tsp Almond Extract
1 tsp Butter Extract
8 packet Sucralose
1/8 tsp Xanthan Gum

Estimated Nutritional Information

Per Cup	
Calories	120.5
Fats	0.5g
Carbs	3g
Protein	26g

Directions

1. Mix all ingredients together in a blender and refrigerate until needed. Stir or shake well before use.

Vegan Version
Replace egg whites with egg white replacement.

Gluten-Free Version
No changes necessary.

Anabolic Milk (Chocolate)

Ingredients

1 cup Egg White
1 tbsp Cocoa Powder
8 packet Sucralose
1/8 tsp Xanthan Gum

Estimated Nutritional Information

Per Cup	
Calories	150
Fats	2g
Carbs	6g
Protein	27g

Directions

1. Mix all ingredients together in a blender and refrigerate until needed. Stir or shake well before use.

Vegan Version
Replace egg whites with egg white replacement.

Gluten-Free Version
No changes necessary.

Anabolic Milk (Coffee Creamer)

Ingredients

1 cup Egg White
1/2 tbsp Mrs Butterworths No Sugar Added Syrup
1/2 tbsp Vanilla Extract
8 packet Sucralose
1/8 tsp Xanthan Gum

Estimated Nutritional Information

Per Cup	
Calories	120.5
Fats	0.5g
Carbs	3g
Protein	26g

Directions

1. Mix all ingredients together in a blender and refrigerate until needed. Stir or shake well before use.

Vegan Version
Replace egg whites with egg white replacement.

Gluten-Free Version
No changes necessary.

Anabolic Milk (Strawberry)

Ingredients

1 cup Egg White
3 Strawberries
8 packet Sucralose
1/8 tsp Xanthan Gum

Estimated Nutritional Information

Per Cup	
Calories	134.5
Fats	0.5g
Carbs	6g
Protein	26.5g

Directions

1. Mix all ingredients together in a blender and refrigerate until needed. Stir or shake well before use.

Vegan Version
Replace egg whites with egg white replacement.

Gluten-Free Version
No changes necessary.

Anabolic Milk (Vanilla)

Ingredients

1 cup Egg White
1 tbsp Vanilla Extract
8 packet Sucralose
1/8 tsp Xanthan Gum

Estimated Nutritional Information

Per Cup	
Calories	120.5
Fats	0.5g
Carbs	3g
Protein	26g

Directions

1. Mix all ingredients together in a blender and refrigerate until needed. Stir or shake well before use.

Vegan Version
Replace egg whites with egg white replacement.

Gluten-Free Version
No changes necessary.

BREAKFAST

Carrot Cake Porridge

Ingredients

1/3 cup Almond Milk
1/3 cup Rolled Oats
1/2 cup Egg Whites
1 packet Cyclamate
2 tsp Cinnamon
1 tsp Nutmeg
1 large OR 2 small Carrots, shredded
1 scoop Vanilla OR Cinnamon Protein Powder
1/4 cup Mrs Butterworths No Sugar Added Syrup

Estimated Nutritional Information

Makes 1 Serving	
Calories	333.5
Fats	3.5g
Carbs	33.5g
Protein	42g

Directions

1. In a medium pot add almond milk, eggs, oats, cyclamate, cinnamon, nutmeg and carrot. If using a cinnamon protein powder use only 1 tsp of cinnamon.
2. Stir constantly with rubber spatula over medium-high heat until mixture thickens up, really scrap the bottom to keep eggs from burning.
3. Remove from heat, stir in protein powder and maple syrup.
4. Let rest to thicken up, stirring occasionally, for 5 minutes.
5. Transfer to bowl, sprinkle on cinnamon or add berries and other toppings if desired.

Vegan Version
Replace egg whites with egg white replacement.

Gluten-Free Version
No changes necessary.

Champion Oatmeal

Ingredients

1/3 cup Water
1/3 cup Rolled Oats
1 scoop Vanilla Protein Powder
1/2 cup Egg Whites
1/4 cup Mrs Butterworths No Sugar Added Syrup
1 packet Cyclamate
(Optional) Diced Apple
(Optional) Cinnamon
(Optional) Berries

Estimated Nutritional Information

Makes 1 Serving
Does not count optionals

Calories	305
Fats	3.5g
Carbs	26.5g
Protein	42g

Directions

1. In a medium pot add water, eggs, oats, cyclamate and apple pieces if using.
2. Stir constantly with rubber spatula over high heat until mixture thickens up, really scrap the bottom to keep eggs from burning.
3. Remove from heat, stir in protein powder and maple syrup.
4. Let rest to thicken up, stirring occasionally, for 5 minutes.
5. Transfer to bowl, sprinkle on cinnamon or add berries and other toppings if desired.

Vegan Version
Replace egg whites with egg white replacement.

Gluten-Free Version
No changes necessary.

French Toast

Ingredients

2 Slices of Bread
1 cup Egg Whites
1/4 cup Almond Milk
1 scoop Protein Powder
2-4 packets Cyclamate
1 tsp Cinnamon
1 tbsp Vanilla
(Optional) Berries or Fruit

Estimated Nutritional Information

Makes 1 Serving 2 Slices of Bread	
Calories	300
Fats	3.5g
Carbs	34.5g
Protein	32.5g

Directions

1. Whisk everything but bread together into a container. You may have clumps depending on the mix-ability of your protein which is fine, they'll dissolve while cooking.
2. Soak pieces of bread in mixture until fully saturated.
3. Cook flipping half way through. If using berries/fruit place them underneath the bread so they cook into it.
   1. Air fry – 180°C/350°F for 8-10 minutes.
   2. Frying Pan – Medium heat until both sides golden brown.
4. Unused mixture can be put in the fridge and used again.

Vegan Version
Replace egg whites with egg white replacement.

Gluten-Free Version
Use gluten-free bread.

Muesli

Ingredients

1/2 cups rolled oats
1/2 cup wheat bran
1/4 cup raw pecans, coarsely chopped
1/2 teaspoon kosher salt
1/2 teaspoon ground cinnamon
1/4 cup dried fruit of choice
1 cup Anabolic Milk

Estimated Nutritional Information

Makes 1 Serving

Calories	474
Fats	10g
Carbs	59g
Protein	37g

Directions

1. Preheat oven to 180°C/350°F.
2. In a large bowl add oats, bran, almonds, and pecans.
3. Very lightly spray with cooking oil.
4. Sprinkle salt and cinnamon over top, toss to coat.
5. Transfer bowl to a cooking sheet.
6. Place on top rack in oven and toast mixture for about 10 minutes.
7. Transfer back to a bowl and add in fruit. Toss to mix.
8. Mixture can be placed into a container for meal prep at this point.
9. When ready to consume, put in bowl and pour a cup of anabolic milk over top.

Vegan Version
Use vegan version of anabolic milk.

Gluten-Free Version
No changes necessary.

Pancake Ala Protein

Ingredients

1/2 cup Egg White or Anabolic Milk (Cake Batter)
1/4 cup Almond Milk
1/2 cup Flour
1/2 tsp Baking Powder
1 packet Cyclamate

Estimated Nutritional Information

Makes 1 Serving Uses Anabolic Milk	
Calories	306
Fats	2g
Carbs	52g
Protein	20g

Directions

1. Spray a pan lightly with cooking spray and place over medium heat, allow to heat up for a couple minutes.
2. Mix all ingredients together into a smooth batter. If too runny, add a little protein powder to thicken it up. Or a little more flour if you have no protein powder.
3. Pour into circles on your pan. Allow to cook until bubbles are popping on the top side then flip. Cook until bottom is golden brown.
4. Stack pancakes, optionally serve with a scoop of Vanilla Protein Frozen Yogurt.

Vegan Version
Use vegan version of anabolic milk.

Gluten-Free Version
Use gluten-free flour.

Protein Breakfast Pudding

Ingredients

1 scoop Vanilla Protein Powder
2 tbsp Psyllium Husk
1 cup Almond Milk
2 packet Cyclamate
1/2 cup Fruit/Berry of Choice

Estimated Nutritional Information

Makes 1 Serving

Calories	182
Fats	4g
Carbs	10g
Protein	26.5g

Directions

1. The night before mix all ingredients in a bowl and set in fridge.
2. In the morning just grab and eat!

Vegan Version
Use vegan protein powder.

Gluten-Free Version
No changes necessary.

Savoury French Toast

Ingredients

2 Slices of Bread
1 1/2 cups Egg Whites
1 tsp Cumin
1 tsp Salt
1 tsp Pepper

Estimated Nutritional Information

Per Serving 2 Pieces of Bread	
Calories	315
Fats	3g
Carbs	26.5g
Protein	45.5g

Directions

1. Pour egg whites into a bowl. Add bread and allow to soak.
2. While bread soaks, prepare a large non-stick pan over medium high heat if using the stove or preheat air fryer to 180°C/350°F.
3. Transfer bread to pan or air fryer.
4. Add salt and pepper to left over egg white and mix.
5. Pour left over egg white onto pan to fry, or into 1-2 egg circles and place in air fryer.
6. Cook
   - On Stove – Until bread is golden brown
   - Air Fryer – At 180°C/350°F for 10 minutes
7. Stack fried egg on top of bread and enjoy.

Vegan Version
Replace egg whites with egg white replacement.

Gluten-Free Version
Use gluten-free bread.

Super Simple Protein Cereal

Ingredients

1 cup Anabolic Milk
1 1/2 cup Cereal

Estimated Nutritional Information

Depends On Cereal Add Anabolic Milk To Cereal	
Calories	-
Fats	-
Carbs	-
Protein	-

Directions

1. Preference goes to high fibre high protein cereals like Kashi Go Lean. But if you have room for carbs you can use any cereal.

Vegan Version
Use vegan version of anabolic milk.

Gluten-Free Version
Use gluten-free cereal.

LUNCH

Croque Monsieur

Ingredients

4 slices Bread, crust removed
1/2 cup Anabolic Milk (Vanilla)
1/2 cup Low Fat Shredded Cheese
1/2 tsp Salt
1/2 tsp Pepper
Pinch of Nutmeg
1 tbsp Dijon Mustard
2 medium Slices of Ham (~40g each)

Directions

1. Preheat oven to 200°C/400°F.
2. In a small pot over low heat, add anabolic milk and stir for 2 minutes.
3. Add cheese to pot and stir until fully melted and incorporated. Remove from heat.
4. Add salt, pepper and nutmeg to pot. Stir and set aside.
5. Place bread on baking sheet and toast in oven for 3 minutes per side.
6. Spread mustard over two slices of bread, cover with slices of ham, then cover with remaining two slices of bread.
7. Pour cheese sauce over both sandwiches.
8. Return to oven and bake for 5 minutes. Then turn on broiler and bake until cheese become golden, 3-5 minutes.
9. Let cool and enjoy.

Vegan Version

Use vegan version of anabolic milk, use vegan cheese, replace ham with vegan deli meat.

Gluten-Free Version

Use gluten-free bread.

Low Carb Ramen

Ingredients

1 package of <u>Konjac Noodles</u> (<u>Alternative</u>)
2 cups No Fat Chicken Broth
2 tsp MSG
2 tsp <u>Poultry Seasoning</u>
2 tsp Onion Powder
2 tsp Garlic Powder
1 Chicken Breast, shredded
1/2 cup Diced Red Cabbage
1/2 cup Diced Carrots
1/2 cup Diced Green Onions

Estimated Nutritional Information

Makes One Serving

Calories	272
Fats	4g
Carbs	26g
Protein	33g

Directions

1. In a medium pot bring chicken broth and soy sauce to a boil over high heat.
2. Turn down heat to medium, add noodles, poultry seasoning, onion powder, garlic powder, chicken, cabbage, carrots and onions and let simmer for 8-10 minutes.
3. Pour into a bowl and serve.

Vegan Version
Replace chicken broth with vegetable broth and chicken with tofu.

Gluten-Free Version
No changes necessary.

IMPORTANT WARNING: CHOKING HAZARD.

Konjac root does not dissolve normally in the mouth like most food, which may cause a choking hazard in young children if not chewed thoroughly. Recipe not recommended for young children.

Meaty Mac & Cheese

Ingredients

1 cup 90% (or more) Lean Ground Beef
1 cup Better Than Pasta Konjac Penne
1/2 cup Low Fat Shredded Cheese
1/4 cup Nonfat Cream Cheese
1/2 cup Almond Milk
2 tsp Dry Mustard
2 tsp Salt

Estimated Nutritional Information

Makes One Serving
Uses 90% Lean Beef

Calories	604
Fats	34g
Carbs	8.5g
Protein	66g

Directions

1. Spray a medium pot with cooking spray and put over medium-high heat.
2. Add beef, 1 tsp mustard and 1 tsp salt. Stir to coat and cook until brown.
3. Remove beef to a bowl and set aside.
4. Add almond milk and konjac penne to pot, heat until it starts to have whisks of steam.
5. Add cream cheese and shredded cheese, whisk until mixed.
6. (Optional) Add beef back in, stir to coat and transfer to bowl.
7. (Optional) Serve pasta over-top bowl of beef.

Vegan Version

Replace ground beef with beyond meat or tofu, shredded cheese with vegan cheese, remove cream cheese.

Gluten-Free Version

No changes necessary.

Protein Cheese Bun

Ingredients

1 Ciabatta Bun
1/2 cup Egg White
1/2 scoop Vanilla Protein Powder
1/2 cup Low-Fat Shredded Cheese

Estimated Nutritional Information

Makes One Serving	
Calories	456.5
Fats	8.5g
Carbs	47g
Protein	48g

Directions

1. Use a knife to cut a cross in the top of the bun
2. Mix egg white and protein powder together.
3. Pour the egg white mixture into scored bun and allow to saturate for a minute.
4. Cook
   - Air Fryer – 180°C/350°F for 10 minutes
   - Oven – 180°C/350°F for 15 minutes
5. Halfway through cooking, remove bun and sprinkle with cheese. Return to oven/air fryer.

Vegan Version
Replace egg white with egg white replacement, cheese with vegan cheese, and use vegan protein powder.

Gluten-Free Version
Use a gluten-free bun.

Pizza Bagel

Ingredients

1 Bagel, halved
1/4 cup Egg White
1/2 cup Low-Fat Cheese
1/4 cup Low Calorie Marinara or Pizza Sauce
(Optional) Turkey Pepperoni
(Optional) Shredded Chicken
(Optional) Pineapple?

Estimated Nutritional Information

Makes One Serving
Does Not Count Optionals

Calories	381.5
Fats	5.5g
Carbs	53g
Protein	30g

Directions

1. Slowly pour the egg white over the two bagel halves, letting it soak in.
2. Spread sauce over bagels.
3. Sprinkle cheese and choice of toppings on top.
4. Cook
   - Oven – 180°C/350°F for 20 minutes
   - Air Fryer – 180°C/350°F for 10 minutes
5. Remove and let cool.

Vegan Version
Replace egg whites with egg replacer. Use a vegan cheese and toppings.

Gluten-Free Version
Use a gluten-free bun.

SUPPER

Air Fried Chicken Fried Steak

Ingredients

1/2 lbs (226g) Cube Steak
1/4 cup Egg White
1/4 cup Flour
1 tsp Garlic Powder
1 tsp Paprika
1 tsp Salt
1/2 tsp Pepper
1/4 cup St. Hubert Dijon Gravy

Estimated Nutritional Information

Makes One Serving

Calories	417
Fats	13g
Carbs	18g
Protein	57g

Directions

1. Use paper towel to absorb excess moisture in steak.
2. In one bowl add egg whites.
3. In second bowl add flour and spices.
4. Coat steak in spice mix, then transfer to egg whites and coat, then back to spice mix for final coat.
5. Cook
   - Air Fry 200°C/400°F for 10 minutes, flipping half way.
6. Top with gravy.

Vegan Version
Replace steak with tofu and egg white with egg white replacement.

Gluten-Free Version
Use gluten-free flour.

Chicken Fried Rice

Ingredients

1 Minute Rice Ready-To-Serve Cup, pre-cooked
1 Chicken Breast
1 cup Egg Whites
1 Shallot, diced
1 clove Garlic, minced
1/4 cup Soy Sauce
1 cup Frozen Veggies

Estimated Nutritional Information

Makes One Serving

Calories	585
Fats	9g
Carbs	60g
Protein	66g

Directions

1. Dice chicken into cubes, sprinkle with salt.
2. Spray non-stick pan with light coat of oil and set over medium-high heat.
3. Add egg whites, folding them as they cook.
4. Remove egg whites to separate bowl.
5. Add shallot and garlic to pan, cook until shallot turns translucent.
6. Add chicken and rice, cook stirring occasionally until chicken is nearly done (~6 minutes)
7. Add frozen veggies and cook for another two minutes.

Vegan Version

Replace chicken with tofu and egg whites with egg replacement

Gluten-Free Version

No changes necessary.

Chili

Ingredients

1 tsp Olive Oil
1 Shallot, Diced
1 cup 98% Lean Ground Beef
2 tsp Cumin
2 tsp Garlic Powder
2 tsp Salt
1 tsp Pepper
1 cup Kidney Beans
1 cup Beef Broth
1 cup No Sugar Added Ketchup

Estimated Nutritional Information

Makes One Serving

Calories	587
Fats	15g
Carbs	45g
Protein	68g

Directions

1. Add oil to a medium pot and put over medium-high heat.
2. Add shallot and cook until translucent and fragrant.
3. Add beef and cook until brown.
4. Add rest of ingredients.
5. Turn heat up to high and bring to boil. After boiling, reduce heat to medium and let simmer until thickened.

Vegan Version

Replace beef with beyond meat or tofu and beef broth with vegetable broth.

Gluten-Free Version

No changes necessary.

Cottage Pie

Ingredients

1 tsp Olive Oil
1 Garlic Clove , minced
1 Onion, Carrot and Celery, diced
1 cup 98% Lean Ground Beef
1 tbsp No Sugar Added Ketchup
1/2 cups Beef Broth
1 tbsp Worcestershire sauce
1 tsp dried thyme
1/2 tsp salt
1/4 tsp black pepper
1/2 medium Potato
1 tbsp Anabolic Milk (Vanilla)

Estimated Nutritional Information

Makes One Serving

Calories	502.5
Fats	14.5g
Carbs	34g
Protein	59g

Directions

1. Add oil to a skillet or pan over medium-high heat. Add onion and garlic and cook for 1 minute. Add carrot and celery and cook 3 minutes.
2. Turn heat up to high and add beef, stirred until browned.
3. Add ketchup, stock, worcestershire sauce, thyme, salt and pepper. Bring to a simmer and turn heat down to medium-high. Cook until reduced to a gravy.
4. Transfer to a small pie tin, for best results allow to cool.
5. Preheat oven to 180°C/350°F.
6. In small pot boil potato for 15 minutes. Drain then return to stove and allow to steam for a minute.
7. Mash potato, adding anabolic milk, until smooth.
8. Spread onto beef mixture, use a fork to rough up surface.
9. Bake for 25 minutes or until top is golden.
10. Let cool and enjoy.

Vegan Version
Replace beef with beyond meat, beef broth with vegetable and use vegan version of anabolic milk.

Gluten-Free Version
No changes necessary.

Low Carb Pho

Ingredients

1 package of Konjac Noodles (Alternative)
4 cups Beef Broth
150g sliced Roast Beef
1 tbsp Fish Sauce
1/2 diced Yellow Onion
1 piece Thinly Slice Ginger
2 Cloves
2 Star Anise
1 Cinnamon Stick
1 cup Bean Sprouts
3 Scallions
1 Lime Wedge

Estimated Nutritional Information

Makes One Serving	
Calories	447
Fats	11g
Carbs	23g
Protein	64g

Directions

1. Bring beef broth to boil. Reduce heat, add fish sauce, onion, ginger, cloves, star anise and cinnamon stick and allow to simmer for 30-45 minutes. Use a cheesecloth bag for the cloves, star anise and cinnamon if you have one to make the next step easier.
2. Remove the cloves, star anise and cinnamon stick.
3. Add the konjac noodles and simmer for another 10 minutes.
4. While that simmers, cut your roast beef into one inch strips. 150g will be roughly 1/5th of a 2lb package of roast beef.
5. Transfer noodles to a bowl and pour enough broth to cover noodles.
6. Top with roast beef strips, bean sprouts, scallions. Garnish with lime wedge and serve.

Vegan Version

Replace beef with vegan deli meat, beef broth with vegetable, remove fish sauce.

Gluten-Free Version

No changes necessary.

IMPORTANT WARNING: CHOKING HAZARD.

Konjac root does not dissolve normally in the mouth like most food, which may cause a choking hazard in young children if not chewed thoroughly. Recipe not recommended for young children.

Poor Man's Lobster

Ingredients

2 Cod Filet
4 cups Diet 7-Up or Sprite
1 cup Unsweetened Apple Sauce

Estimated Nutritional Information	
Makes One Serving One Serving is Two Fillets	
Calories	477
Fats	3g
Carbs	30g
Protein	82.5g

Directions

1. Pour diet soda into pot and bring to boil.
2. Add cod, cooking for roughly 10 minutes until filets are nice and flakey.
3. Remove and plate, use apple sauce for dipping instead of butter.

Vegan Version
Sorry vegans, nothing you can do on this one.

Gluten-Free Version
No changes necessary.

Power Potatoes

Ingredients

1/2 Chicken Breast, cubed
1 medium Potato, diced
1 tsp Sea Salt
1/2 tsp Black Pepper
1 tsp Chili Sauce
1 tsp Garlic Powder
1/2 tsp Paprika
4 tbsp Low-fat Cottage Cheese
2 tsp chopped Chives
1/2 cup Low-Fat Shredded Cheese

Estimated Nutritional Information

Makes One Serving

Calories	387
Fats	7g
Carbs	44g
Protein	37g

Directions

1. Preheat oven to 200°C/400°F.
2. Mix chicken, potato, salt, pepper, chili sauce, garlic powder and paprika in bowl, then transfer to small casserole dish or baking pan.
3. Place in oven for 30 minutes.
4. Remove from oven, stir in cottage cheese and place back in oven for 25 minutes.
5. Remove from oven, sprinkle shredded cheese and chives over potatoes and place back in over for about 5 minutes until cheese is melted.
6. Remove, let cool and enjoy.

Vegan Version

Replace chicken with tofu, remove cottage cheese and use shredded vegan cheese.

Gluten-Free Version

No changes necessary.

Smokey Beans And Baked Eggs

Ingredients

2 tsp Olive Oil
1 Shallot, diced
1 Red Pepper, sliced into strips
1 Garlic Clove, crushed
1 tsp Smoked Paprika
5.5oz (150ml) can Tomato Paste
1 cup Black Beans
1/2 cup Egg White

Estimated Nutritional Information

Makes One Serving

Calories	565
Fats	13g
Carbs	75g
Protein	37g

Directions

1. If using dry beans, soak over night then dispose of water. If used canned beans, drain water.
2. In a pan with a lid, heat olive oil over medium high heat.
3. Add shallot and cook stirring frequently until soft and fragrant.
4. Add red pepper and cook for 5 minutes until soft.
5. Add garlic, paprika, and tomatoes. Stir then cover with lid and let simmer over medium heat for 10 minutes.
6. Stir in beans. Make a small hole in the middle of the mixture to see the bottom of the pan and pour egg whites in.
7. Cover and let cook over low heat for 5 minutes until egg whites are cooked.

Vegan Version
Replace egg whites with egg white replacement.

Gluten-Free Version
No changes necessary.

Spring Roll

Ingredients

Spring Roll Wrappers
2 Garlic Cloves , chopped
1 Chicken Breast, diced
1 1/2 cups diced Mushroom
1 1/2 cups Shredded Carrot
1 1/2 cups Bean Sprouts
1 1/2 cups Shredded Cabbage
1 tsp Cornstarch
1 1/2 tbsp Oyster Sauce
2 tsp Soy Sauce
1 tbsp Egg White or Water

Estimated Nutritional Information

Makes One Serving
Assumes Two Spring Rolls

Calories	478
Fats	6g
Carbs	60g
Protein	46g

Directions

1. Spray a non-stick pan lightly with oil and place on stove over high heat.
2. Add garlic and chicken, cooking until chicken is white.
3. Add mushrooms and vegetables and cook for a further 3 minutes.
4. Add cornstarch, oyster sauce and soy sauce. Cook until liquid is gone.
5. Remove from heat and let cool.
6. Place spring roll wrapper down in a diamond shape, place handful of mixture onto one end. Roll mixture half-way, then fold in edges and continue rolling the rest of the way. Use a dab of egg white or water on the final corner before rolling to create a seal.
7. Cook
   - Air Fryer – 180°C/350°F for 13 minutes
   - Oven – 180°C/350°F for 25 minutes
8. Enjoy with a low calorie dip.

Vegan Version
Replace chicken with tofu, remove oyster sauce.

Gluten-Free Version
Use gluten-free spring roll wrappers.

Stuffed Pepper

Ingredients

1 tsp Olive Oil
1 cup 98% Lean Ground Beef
1 Shallot, diced
1 Garlic Clove, minced
1/2 tsp Salt
1/4 tsp Pepper
5.5oz (150ml) can Tomato Paste
1/2 tsp Cumin
1 Minute Rice Ready-To-Serve Cup
2 Large Green Pepper
1/2 cup Low-Fat Shredded Cheese

Estimated Nutritional Information

Makes One Serving
One Serving is Two Peppers

Calories	602
Fats	18g
Carbs	63g
Protein	47g

Directions

1. Preheat oven to 180°C/350°F.
2. In a small pot over medium-high heat add the olive oil and shallot, cook stirring occasionally until it starts to soften.
3. Add the ground beef, garlic, salt and pepper. Cook stirring and breaking up the meat until browned.
4. Add the tomato paste, cumin and minute rice (do not need to microwave it first). Cover pot and let cook for 5 minutes, occasionally stirring to break up the rice.
5. Set a large pot of water on stove to boil.
6. Prepare your green peppers by cutting the top off and spooning out the seeds. Place in a large pot of water and boil for 4 minutes.
7. Remove and drain peppers on paper towel. Fill with stuffing mixture, any excess mixture just place in baking pan. Stand up in baking pan (cut the bottom flat if you need to) and cover with tinfoil. Bake for 30 minutes.
8. Remove from oven, uncover and sprinkle cheese on top. Return to oven and bake another 15-20 minutes until cheese is lightly browned.

Vegan Version

Replace beef with beyond meat and cheese with vegan cheese.

Gluten-Free Version

No changes necessary.

SNACKS

Berry Proteinous Milkshake

Ingredients

2 cups Anabolic Milk
2 scoops Protein Frozen Yogurt
1 cup Berry of Choice or Mixed Berries

Estimated Nutritional Information

Makes One Serving	
Calories	478.5
Fats	2.5g
Carbs	40g
Protein	74g

Directions

1. Place all ingredients into a blender and blend until frothy.
2. If you want it thicker, add up to 1/2 tsp of xanthan gum.

Vegan Version
Use vegan version of anabolic milk and frozen yogurt.

Gluten-Free Version
No changes necessary.

Caramel Protein Popcorn

Ingredients

1 bag Orville Reddenbacher Smart Pop Popcorn
OR
8 cups Air Popped Popcorn
1/2 cup Egg White
2 tsp Caramel Flavour
1/2 tsp Xanthan Gum
1/2 tsp Baking Powder

Estimated Nutritional Information

Makes One Serving

Calories	312
Fats	4g
Carbs	48g
Protein	21g

Directions

1. Pop your popcorn and transfer to a large bowl.
2. Blend egg white, caramel flavour, xanthan gum and baking powder. Let stand for a minute to let the xanthan gum absorb moisture then blend again.
3. Pour mixture over popcorn. Use a spatula to fold the popcorn until mixture is evenly coated.
4. Options:
   - Eat as is.
   - Place in freezer until mixture solidifies.
   - Transfer to baking pan and bake in oven at 250oF for 20-30 minutes, taking it out to mix every 10 minutes.

Vegan Version
Replace egg whites with egg white replacement.

Gluten-Free Version
No changes necessary.

Muffin

Ingredients

3 tbsp Protein Powder
1/4 cup Mrs Butterworths No Sugar Added Syrup
3 tbsp Flour
2 tbsp Psyllium Husk
1 tsp Baking Powder
1 packet Cyclamate
Water

Estimated Nutritional Information

Makes One Serving	
Calories	249
Fats	1.5g
Carbs	44g
Protein	15g

Directions

1. Add all ingredients together in a bowl except water and mix.
2. Add water 1 tbsp at a time as needed to mixture until it becomes a batter consistency, this will change depending on the protein powder used.
3. Spoon mixture into a silicone cupcake mold.
4. Bake
   - Oven – 180°C/350°F for 20-25 minutes.
   - Air Fryer – 180°C/350°F for 12 minutes.
5. Let cool and enjoy.

Vegan Version
Use vegan protein powder.

Gluten-Free Version
Use gluten-free flour.

Protein Cookie

Ingredients

1 scoop Vanilla Protein Powder
1 tbsp Powdered Peanut Butter
2 tbsp Flour
4 packet Cyclamate
1 tsp Baking Soda
2 tbsp Egg White
1/4 cup Mrs Butterworths No Sugar Added Syrup
1/8 cup Sugar Free Chocolate Chips
Almond Milk

Estimated Nutritional Information

Calories Are For Entire Dough Divide By Amount Made

Calories	362
Fats	10g
Carbs	34g
Protein	34g

Directions

1. Mix all ingredients except almond milk together.
2. If mix is too dry, slowly add almond milk to achieve a cookie dough consistency.
3. Move dough to baking sheet or air fryer.
4. Cook
   - Oven – 180°C/350°F for 20 minutes.
   - Air Fryer – 180°C/350°F for 10 minutes.
5. Remove and let cool before eating.

Vegan Version

Use vegan protein powder, replace egg white with egg replacer and add an extra 1 tsp baking soda.

Gluten-Free Version

Use gluten-free flour.

Protein Egg White Chips

Ingredients

1 cup Egg White
1/4 cup Psyllium Husk
2 tsp Popcorn Seasoning

Estimated Nutritional Information

Makes One Serving	
Calories	294.5
Fats	0.5g
Carbs	44g
Protein	28.5g

Directions

1. Mix egg whites and psyllium husk.
2. Lightly coat a 11x15" baking pan with oil.
3. Spread mixture over pan to form a thin coat.
4. Cook in oven at 180°C/350°F for roughly 15 minutes until no longer liquidy.
5. Remove from oven and carefully (warning: hot) rip into bite sized pieces.
6. Place back in oven for roughly 30 minutes until nice and crispy (depends on how thin the mixture spread).
7. Remove from oven and put pieces in a bowl, lightly spray with oil and toss with popcorn seasoning.

Vegan Version
Replace egg white with egg white replacement.

Gluten-Free Version
No changes necessary.

Protein Fudge

Ingredients

1 cup Anabolic Milk (Chocolate)
2 scoops Chocolate Protein Powder
8 packet Sucralose
4 tbsp Psyllium Husk Powder

Estimated Nutritional Information

**Calories For One Batch
Divide by Amount of Pieces**

Calories	520
Fats	4g
Carbs	44g
Protein	77g

Directions

1. Mix all ingredients together in bowl.
2. Transfer mix to silicone mold.
3. Freeze until firm.

Vegan Version
Use vegan version of anabolic milk and a vegan protein powder.

Gluten-Free Version
No changes necessary.

Protein Peanut Butter Bars

Ingredients

Base
6 cups Cheerios
1 1/3 cup Anabolic Milk (Vanilla)

Filling
1 cup Anabolic Milk (Vanilla)
2 cup Powdered Peanut Butter
5 packet Sucralose

Icing
1 cup Walden Farm's Zero Calorie Chocolate Syrup

Estimated Nutritional Information

Calories Per Batch Divide by Amount of Bars	
Calories	1909
Fats	37g
Carbs	224g
Protein	170g

Directions

1. Preheat oven 325°F/160°C
2. Put Cheerios in a blender and blast with a couple quick pulses to break them into chunks.
3. In a medium bowl mix blended Cheerios with 1 1/3 cup anabolic milk into a dough like consistency.
4. Lightly spray a 8"x8" (20cm x 20cm) pan with cooking spray and transfer base mixture to pan. Press flat and place in oven for 15 minutes.
5. In your medium bowl, add all the filling ingredients and mix. When the base has cooked 15 minutes, remove it and cover with the filling mixture. Place back in the oven for 15 minutes.
6. Pour chocolate syrup over filling and set in fridge to cool.

Vegan Version
Use vegan version of anabolic milk.

Gluten-Free Version
No changes necessary.

Vanilla Protein Frozen Yogurt

Ingredients

1 cup No-Fat Greek Yogurt
1 scoop Vanilla Protein
1 tbsp Vanilla Extract
1 tbsp Erythritol
1/4 cup Mrs Butterworths No Sugar Added Syrup

Estimated Nutritional Information

Makes One Serving	
Calories	295
Fats	1.5g
Carbs	32.5g
Protein	47g

Directions

1. Mix all ingredients together in bowl.
2. Place in freezer until scoop-able, roughly 4-6 hours.
3. If over-frozen, allow to thaw before scooping.
4. Can be transferred to fridge for an hour once it's in the scoop-able stage.

Vegan Version

Use soy yogurt (will have a lot less protein though) and vegan protein powder.

Gluten-Free Version

No changes necessary.

Need more recipes?

Want to learn how nutrition works?

Want an honest overview of supplements?

Make sure you check out my Nutrition Guide

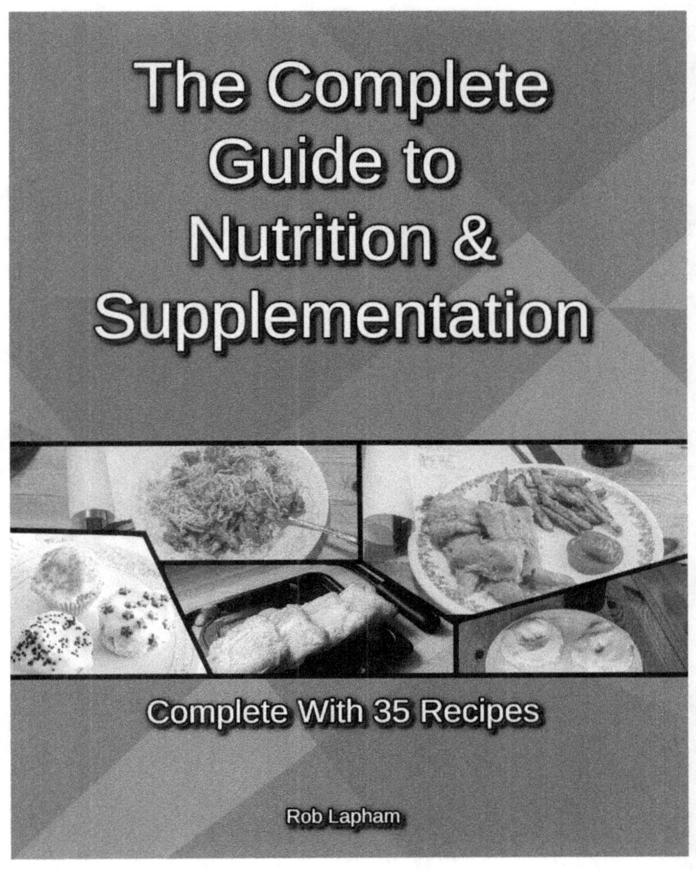